# Understanding Binge Eating Disorder

## Causes, Symptoms, Treatment, and Recovery

By

## George J. Rosen

# Table of Content

# Introduction

A kind of eating disorder known as binge eating disorder (BED) is defined by recurrent episodes in which a person consumes a lot of food quickly and feels like they have no control over their eating. Individuals with BED often experience guilt, shame, and distress after bingeing, leading to a vicious cycle of bingeing and emotional distress.

Below are some essential details regarding binge eating disorders:

**Prevalence**: BED is the most common eating disorder in the United States, affecting 2–3% of the general population. Women experience it more often than men do.

**Causes:** Although the precise origins of BED are not yet entirely known, it is thought to be a complex interplay of genetic, biological, psychological, and social factors. Some common risk factors for developing BED include a history of dieting, low self-esteem, depression, and a family history of eating disorders.

**Symptoms:** The hallmark symptom of BED is binge eating, characterized by consuming an abnormally large amount of food in a short time, often to the point of discomfort. Other symptoms may include:

- Eating rapidly.
- Eating alone due to embarrassment.
- Feeling guilty, ashamed, or depressed after bingeing.

Consequences: BED can lead to various physical and emotional effects, including weight gain, obesity, gastrointestinal problems, diabetes, high blood pressure, and depression. It can also hurt social functioning and quality of life.

**Treatment:** BED is treatable, and several evidence-based interventions are effective, including cognitive-behavioral therapy (CBT), interpersonal therapy (IPT), and medication. Treatment may involve a combination of approaches, and it is vital to work with a trained healthcare professional to develop an individualized treatment plan.

**Self-help:** In addition to seeking professional treatment, there are also several self-help strategies that individuals with BED can try, such as developing a regular eating schedule, practicing mindful eating, and engaging in regular physical activity. It is essential to seek support from loved ones and to practice self-compassion and self-care.

# Chapter 1:

# Introduction

Binge eating disorder (BED) is a complex and severe mental health condition affecting millions worldwide. It is characterized by recurrent episodes of consuming large amounts of food quickly and often feeling uncomfortably full or experiencing physical discomfort. Individuals with BED usually experience a sense of loss of control over their eating during these episodes and may feel guilty, ashamed, or distressed afterward.

As a specific diagnosis, BED is a clinically A disorder acknowledged in the Diagnostic and Statistical Manual of Mental Disorders (DSM-5). In the United States, it is the most prevalent eating disorder, affecting an estimated 2–3% of the general population and being more common in women than men.

If left untreated, BED can have significant physical, emotional, and social consequences. It can lead to weight gain, obesity, gastrointestinal problems, diabetes, high blood pressure, and depression. It can also hurt social functioning and quality of life.

Fortunately, BED is treatable, and several evidence-based interventions have been shown, including cognitive-behavioral therapy (CBT), interpersonal therapy (IPT), dialectical behavior therapy (DBT), and medication.

Treatment may involve a combination of approaches, and it is essential to work with a trained healthcare professional to develop an individualized treatment plan.

This book aims to comprehensively understand BED, including its causes, symptoms, and treatment options. It will also highlight personal stories of recovery and provide resources and references for individuals with BED and their loved ones. By increasing awareness and understanding of BED, we hope to support individuals in their journey toward recovery and improved well-being.

## Definition of binge eating disorder (BED)

Binge eating disorder (BED), as an eating disorder, is characterized by binge eating, which is distinguished by repetitive instances of consuming large quantities of food within a brief period, often accompanied by a sense of lacking control over one's eating habits. Individuals with BED usually experience guilt, shame, and distress after bingeing, which can lead to a vicious cycle of bingeing and emotional distress. As a specific diagnosis, BED is a clinical disorder acknowledged in the Diagnostic and Statistical Manual of Mental Disorders (DSM-5). If left untreated, it is a severe mental health condition with significant physical, emotional, and social consequences.

## Prevalence and demographics

Binge eating disorder (BED) is the most prevalent in the United States, affecting 2–3 percent of the general population. The likelihood of women having this is higher than that of men, with women making up approximately 60% of individuals with BED. However, research suggests that BED may be underdiagnosed in men due to societal expectations of body image and the stigmatization of eating disorders in men.

BED can affect individuals of any age, but the onset of this disorder typically occurs in late adolescence or early adulthood. Research suggests that individuals with a higher body mass index (BMI) and those who have experienced weight-related stigma are at greater risk for developing BED. Additionally, individuals with a history of dieting, low self-esteem, anxiety, or depression may be more likely to develop BED.

BED also disproportionately affects specific populations, including those with a history of trauma, such as physical or sexual abuse, and individuals who identify as LGBTQ+. Individuals who experience weight-related discrimination or bullying may also be at greater risk of developing BED.

It is important to note that while BED is most commonly diagnosed in individuals who are overweight or obese, not all individuals with BED are overweight or have a high BMI. Furthermore, weight stigma and discrimination can exacerbate the negative psychological and physical consequences of BED, highlighting the need for a comprehensive and individualized approach to treatment.

# Historical background

The concept of binge eating as a clinical phenomenon has been recognized for over a century, with early reports dating back to the late 1800s. Binge eating was identified as an independent eating disorder from anorexia nervosa and bulimia nervosa only during the 1950s and 1960s.

The term "binge eating disorder" (BED) was first used in the 1990s to describe a pattern of binge eating not accompanied by compensatory behaviors such as purging or excessive exercise, characteristic of bulimia nervosa. In 1994, BED was included in the DSM-IV as a provisional diagnosis, meaning it was recognized as a distinct disorder but required further research to establish diagnostic criteria.

The DSM-5 recognized BED as a unique eating disorder in 2013, defining it as repeated instances of binge eating accompanied by a feeling of inability to control eating and providing specific diagnostic criteria. Including BED as a particular diagnosis in the DSM-5 was an essential step toward increasing awareness and recognition of the disorder and improving access to appropriate treatment for those affected.

Over the past several decades, BED research has increased significantly, leading to a greater understanding of the disorder's causes, consequences, and treatment. Nonetheless, there is still much to be discovered about BED, particularly how it intersects with other mental health conditions and individuals from diverse backgrounds. Ongoing research and advocacy efforts are crucial in addressing BED's complex and multifaceted nature.

# Chapter 2:

# Causes and Risk Factors

The origins of binge eating disorder (BED) are multifaceted and can be impacted by several factors. Research suggests that comic, biological, environmental, and psychological factors may cause BED.

One potential biological factor is dysregulation of the reward system in the brain, which may make individuals with BED more susceptible to overeating in response to food cues. Additionally, genetic factors may predispose individuals to BED. However, the specific genes involved have not yet been to environmental factors, such as childhood trauma or adverse life events, which may also contribute to the development of BED. Research has demonstrated that children who have experienced childhood abuse or neglect are at a higher risk of developing BED, potentially due to the emotional dysregulation and maladaptive coping strategies resulting from early trauma.

Psychological factors, such as negative body image, low self-esteem, and perfectionism, may also play a role in the development of BED. Dieting and restrictive eating patterns can also contribute to the development of BED, as these behaviors can lead to increased food cravings and a loss of control over eating.

Certain risk factors may increase an individual's likelihood of developing BED, including a history of dieting or weight cycling, weight stigma or discrimination, and having a relative with an eating disorder or other mental health condition. Additionally, BED is more commonly diagnosed in women, although research suggests it may be underdiagnosed in men.

It's worth emphasizing that these factors can heighten the likelihood of someone developing BED; not everyone who experiences these risk factors will develop the disorder. BED is a complex and multifaceted condition, and the causes and risk factors may vary from person to person. BED treatment should be individualized and address each individual's unique needs and experiences.

## Biological factors

Research suggests biological factors may contribute to developing binge eating disorder (BED). These factors include dysregulation of the reward system in the brain, abnormalities in hunger and satiety signaling, and alterations in brain chemistry.

One potential biological factor contributing to BED is the brain's dysregulation of the reward system. This process entails the discharge of dopamine, a neurotransmitter that has a critical function in the sensation of enjoyment and gratification.

Individuals with BED may have alterations in this system that make them more susceptible to overeating in response to food cues, leading to a loss of control over eating.

Another potential biological factor is abnormalities in hunger and satiety signaling. Hormones such as leptin, ghrelin, and insulin play essential roles in regulating hunger and satiety, and alterations in these hormones may contribute to the development of BED. For example, some studies have suggested that individuals with BED may have lower levels of leptin, a hormone that signals the brain to decrease hunger and increase energy expenditure.

Finally, alterations in brain chemistry may also contribute to the development of BED. Research has shown that individuals with BED may have differences in brain activity and neurotransmitter function compared to individuals without the disorder. For example, some studies have suggested that individuals with BED may have lower serotonin levels, a neurotransmitter crucial in regulating mood and appetite.

While these biological factors may contribute to the development of BED, it is essential to note that they do not necessarily cause the disorder alone. BED is a complex and multifaceted condition, and the interplay between biological, psychological, and environmental factors likely contributes to its development.

## Psychological factors

Psychological factors play a significant role in developing binge eating disorder (BED). These factors can include negative body image, low self-esteem, perfectionism, and difficulties with emotion regulation.

Negative body image is a common psychological factor in BED, and individuals with the disorder may have distorted perceptions of their body size or shape. This can lead to an increased focus on weight and shape, contributing to the development of restrictive eating patterns and dieting behaviors.

Low self-esteem is another psychological factor that may contribute to the development of BED. Individuals with low self-esteem may feel a sense of shame or guilt around their eating behaviors, which can further contribute to feelings of loss of control over eating.

Perfectionism is another psychological factor that may contribute to the development of BED. Individuals with BED may set unattainable standards for themselves, leading to a cycle of perfectionistic thinking and subsequent binge eating to cope with feelings of failure or inadequacy.

Difficulties with emotion regulation are also common in individuals with BED. Such challenges may involve problems recognizing and communicating emotions and a tendency to employ food to manage negative emotions.

It is worth knowing that psychological factors may influence the development of BED, but they are not necessarily the sole cause of the disorder. BED is a complex condition that likely involves the interplay between biological, psychological, and environmental factors. BED treatment should address the unique psychological needs of each individual and help them develop healthier coping strategies for managing emotions and regulating eating behaviors.

## Social and environmental factors

Social and environmental factors are essential in developing binge eating disorder (BED). These factors include social pressure to conform to specific body standards, cultural attitudes towards food and body image, family history of eating disorders, and stressful life events.

Social pressure to conform to specific body standards is a common environmental factor that can contribute to the development of BED. For example, the thin ideal portrayed in media and advertising can lead to feelings of body dissatisfaction and an increased focus on weight and shape. This can contribute to developing restrictive eating patterns and dieting behaviors, which may lead to binge eating.

Cultural attitudes towards food and body image can also influence the development of BED. For example, cultural perspectives promoting restrictive eating and weight loss may contribute to developing disordered eating behaviors, including binge eating.

A family history of eating disorders is another environmental factor that may increase the risk of developing BED. Research suggests that individuals with a family history of eating disorders may be more likely to develop disordered eating behaviors, including binge eating.

Stressful life events, such as trauma, abuse, or significant life changes, can also contribute to the development of BED. These events can trigger emotional distress and lead to the use of food as a coping mechanism. Additionally, stressful events can disrupt standard eating patterns and increase the likelihood of binge eating behaviors.

It's worth emphasizing that these factors can heighten the likelihood of someone developing BED, but they are not necessarily the sole cause of the disorder. BED is a complex condition that likely involves the interplay between biological, psychological, and environmental factors. BED treatment should address the unique social and ecological factors contributing to the disorder and help individuals develop healthier coping strategies for managing stress and regulating eating behaviors.

**Intersectionality and cultural considerations**

Intersectionality and cultural considerations are important when understanding and treating binge eating disorder (BED). BED affects individuals of all races, ethnicities, genders, and socioeconomic backgrounds, but it can present differently depending on a person's cultural experiences and identities.

Intersectionality refers to how different aspects of a person's identity, such as race, gender, sexuality, and class, intersect and interact to shape their experiences and identities.

It is essential to consider intersectionality when working with individuals with BED, as different cultural factors may impact the development and treatment of the disorder.

Cultural considerations are also important when understanding and treating BED. Different cultures may have different attitudes towards food, body image, and eating behaviors, which can impact the disorder's development and maintenance. For example, some cultures may emphasize family meals or traditional foods, while others may prioritize thinness and restrictive eating behaviors.

In addition, cultural factors may impact how BED is perceived and diagnosed. For example, individuals from certain cultures may be more likely to present with atypical symptoms of BED, such as binge eating culturally specific foods or in response to cultural stressors.

It is essential for healthcare providers to approach the treatment of BED with cultural sensitivity and to consider the unique cultural factors that may be impacting an individual's experience with the disorder. Treatment should be tailored to the individual's cultural background and incorporate their beliefs and values around food and body image.

Overall, understanding the intersectionality and cultural considerations of BED is essential for providing effective and culturally sensitive care to individuals with the disorder.

# Chapter 3:

# Symptoms and Diagnosis

The symptoms and diagnosis standards for binge eating disorder (BED) adhere to the Diagnostic and Statistical Manual of Mental Disorders (DSM-5) criteria, fifth edition. To be diagnosed with BED, an individual must meet the following requirements:

**Recurrent episodes of binge eating:** The individual must have recurrent episodes of binge eating, characterized by consuming a substantial quantity of food within a brief duration (e.g., within two hours) while experiencing a sense of loss of control over eating.

Binge-eating disorders are linked with three or more of the subsequent symptoms:

1. Consuming food much quicker than usual
2. Eating until one experience discomfort or pain due to fullness
3. Ingesting vast quantities of food despite not feeling hungry
4. Eating alone as a result of being ashamed of the amount of food consumed
5. Feeling intense self-disgust, depression, or overwhelming guilt after overeating.

Episodes of binge eating transpire at a minimum frequency of once per week over three months.

**Absence of inappropriate compensatory behaviors:** The individual does not engage in inappropriate compensatory behaviors (such as purging, fasting, or excessive exercise) to counteract the binge eating episodes.

**Significant distress or impairment:** The binge eating episodes and associated distress or impairment cannot be more satisfactorily accounted for by another psychological condition, such as bulimia nervosa, anorexia nervosa binge/purge subtype, or avoidant/restrictive food intake disorder.

To diagnose BED, a healthcare professional will typically conduct a comprehensive assessment that includes a physical exam, medical history, and a mental health evaluation. They may also use standardized questionnaires and screening tools to help assess the severity of binge eating behavior and associated symptoms.

It is important to note that BED can be a severe and potentially life-threatening disorder. It is essential to seek professional help from a mental health provider or eating disorder specialist If you or someone you know is displaying symptoms of BED. Early diagnosis and treatment can improve outcomes and reduce the risk of long-term health complications.

**Binge eating behavior and characteristics.**

Binge eating behavior is the hallmark of binge eating disorder (BED). It is characterized by quickly consuming a large amount of food, typically within two hours. During a binge episode, individuals may feel a lack of control over their eating and may continue eating even when physically uncomfortable.

Some common characteristics of binge eating behavior in BED include:

Eating large amounts of food: During a binge episode, individuals may consume much more than most people in a similar situation.

**Rapid eating:** Binge eating episodes typically involve devouring food without regard for hunger or fullness cues.

**Eating in secret:** Individuals with BED may feel ashamed of their binge eating behavior and may try to hide it from others.

**Eating when not physically hungry:** Binge episodes may be triggered by emotional distress, boredom, or other non-physical cues.

**Feeling out of control:** Individuals with BED may feel unable to stop eating during a binge episode, even when they want to.

**Emotional distress:** Binge eating behavior is often accompanied by feelings of guilt, shame, and anxiety.

It's essential to recognize that not everyone who engages in binge eating behavior has BED. Binge eating can also be a symptom of other eating disorders, such as bulimia nervosa or anorexia nervosa binge/purge subtype. Additionally, some individuals may engage in occasional episodes of binge eating without meeting the diagnostic criteria for BED.

Suppose you are concerned about your binge eating behavior or the binge eating behavior of a loved one. In that case, seeking professional help from a mental health provider or eating disorder specialist is essential. BED treatment typically involves a combination of psychotherapy, medication, and nutritional counseling.

## Physical and psychological symptoms

Binge eating disorder (BED) can have a wide range of physical and psychological symptoms, varying in severity depending on the individual. Some of the most common physical and psychological symptoms of BED include:

- Physical symptoms:
- Rapid weight gain or obesity
- Digestive issues, such as bloating, constipation, or diarrhea
- Insomnia or other sleep disturbances
- Fatigue or lethargy
- Joint pain or other musculoskeletal problems
- High blood pressure, high cholesterol, or other cardiovascular problems
- Diabetes or other metabolic disorders
- Psychological symptoms:
- Depression or anxiety
- Low self-esteem or poor body image
- Shame, guilt, or embarrassment
- Social isolation or withdrawal
- Difficulty concentrating or making decisions
- Mood swings or irritability
- Substance abuse or other addictive behaviors

Not everyone with BED will experience all these symptoms, which can vary widely from person to person. Some of these symptoms may also be present in other eating disorders or mental health conditions. A comprehensive evaluation by a mental health professional or eating disorder specialist is necessary to make an accurate diagnosis.

If you or someone you know is undergoing the experience of symptoms associated with BED, seeking professional help from a mental health provider or eating disorder specialist is essential. Early intervention and treatment can improve outcomes and reduce the risk of long-term health complications.

**Diagnostic criteria and assessment tools**

Binge eating disorder (BED) is characterized by recurrent episodes of consuming a considerable amount of food quickly and a sense of loss of control and distress. The diagnostic criteria and assessment tools of BED are as follows:

Diagnostic Criteria:

The diagnostic criteria for BED are outlined as follows:

a) Recurrent episodes of binge eating: The individual must have recurrent episodes of binge eating, characterized by eating a large amount of food in a short period (e.g., within two hours) while experiencing a sense of loss of control over eating.

b) During the episode, an individual experiences a loss of control over eating, such as being unable to stop eating or manage the quantity and type of food consumed. Binge-eating episodes are accompanied by three or more of the following symptoms:

a) Consuming food much quicker than usual

b) Eating until one experiences discomfort or pain due to fullness

c) Ingesting vast quantities of food despite not feeling hungry

d) Eating alone as a result of being ashamed of the amount of food consumed

e) Feeling intense self-disgust, depression, or overwhelming guilt after overeating.

Marked distress regarding binge eating.

Binge eating episodes happen at least once per week, on average, for three months.

**Assessment Tools:**

There are several assessment tools available for BED, including:

**Eating Disorder Examination (EDE):** A semi-structured interview designed to assess the specific features of eating disorders, including BED.

Binge Eating Scale (BES): A self-report questionnaire that assesses the severity of binge eating behaviors.

**Yale-Brown-Cornell Eating Disorders Scale (YBC-EDS):** A semi-structured interview that assesses the presence and severity of various eating disorder symptoms, including binge eating.

**Eating Disorder Inventory (EDI):** is a self-report questionnaire that assesses various symptoms and behaviors associated with eating disorders, including binge eating.

**Questionnaire on Eating and Weight Patterns (QEWP):** A self-report questionnaire that assesses the frequency and severity of various eating disorder symptoms, including binge eating.

It is important to note that the assessment and diagnosis of BED should be conducted by a qualified healthcare professional, such as a licensed psychologist or psychiatrist.

# Chapter 4:

# Consequences of BED

Binge eating disorder (BED) can have a wide range of physical, psychological, and social consequences that can significantly impact an individual's quality of life. Some of the most common effects of BED include:

- Physical consequences:
- Obesity or rapid weight gain
- High blood pressure, high cholesterol, or other cardiovascular problems
- Type 2 diabetes or other metabolic disorders
- Digestive issues, such as bloating, constipation, or diarrhea
- Joint pain or other musculoskeletal problems
- Sleep apnea or other sleep disturbances
- Psychological consequences:
- Depression, anxiety, or other mood disorders
- Low self-esteem or poor body image
- Shame, guilt, or embarrassment
- Social isolation or withdrawal
- Difficulty concentrating or making decisions
- Substance abuse or other addictive behaviors
- Social consequences:
- 

- Strained or damaged relationships with friends, family, or romantic partners
- Difficulty functioning in social or work settings
- Reduced ability to participate in social activities or events
- Negative impact on educational or professional opportunities

It is important to acknowledge that BED can manifest in different ways among individuals and may be influenced by various factors, including the severity and duration of the disorder, the individual's overall health status, and the presence of co-occurring mental health or medical conditions. Early intervention and treatment can help to mitigate the negative consequences of BED and improve long-term outcomes for affected individuals.

**Physical health consequences**

Binge eating disorder (BED) can have a range of physical health consequences, some of which include:

**Obesity or rapid weight gain**: Binge eating often leads to excessive calorie intake, which can result in significant weight gain and obesity. This, in turn, can increase the risk of developing various health problems, such as cardiovascular disease, type 2 diabetes, and high blood pressure.

**Cardiovascular problems:** The likelihood of cardiovascular complications, such as heart disease, stroke, and elevated cholesterol levels, may be heightened by obesity and weight gain.

**Type 2 diabetes:** Binge eating disorder can increase the risk of developing type 2 diabetes, particularly in individuals who are overweight or obese. Diabetes can cause various health problems, such as nerve damage, blindness, and kidney disease.

**Digestive issues**: Binge eating can cause digestive problems, such as bloating, constipation, or diarrhea. In more extreme situations, it may also result in gastrointestinal complications, such as bowel obstruction or perforation.

**Joint pain or musculoskeletal problems:** Excessive weight gain associated with binge eating can place additional strain on the joints, leading to joint pain or other musculoskeletal problems.

**Sleep apnea:** People with BED are at increased risk of developing sleep apnea, a sleep disorder characterized by breathing interruptions during sleep. This can result in poor-quality sleep, fatigue, and an increased risk of accidents. It is important to note that these physical health consequences can vary in severity depending on the duration and severity of the binge eating disorder and the individual's overall health status.

Seeking treatment and support can help manage these physical health consequences and improve overall health and well-being.

## Psychological and emotional consequences

Binge eating disorder (BED) can also have psychological and emotional consequences, impacting an individual's quality of life. Some of these consequences include the following:

**Depression and anxiety:** People with BED often experience depression, anxiety, or other mood disorders, which feelings of shame g self-esteem can trigger.

**Low self-esteem and poor body image:** Binge eating can lead to weight gain, contributing to low self-esteem and negative body image. This can lead to avoidance of social situations and increased isolation.

**Shame and guilt:** People with BED often feel ashamed or guilty about their eating behaviors, which can further exacerbate their emotional distress and lead to isolation.

**Impaired cognitive function:** Binge eating can impair cognitive function, leading to difficulty concentrating or making decisions.

**Substance abuse or other addictive behaviors:** People with BED may turn to substances or other addictive behaviors, such as alcohol or drugs, to cope with their emotional distress.

**Social isolation:** People with BED may avoid social situations or withdraw from relationships due to shame or fear of judgment.

**Eating disorders and comorbid mental health conditions:** Binge eating disorder frequently co-occurs with other eating disorders, such as bulimia nervosa or anorexia nervosa. Additionally, it may be accompanied by other psychological conditions such as anxiety and depression.

It is essential to seek BED treatment, as untreated BED can lead to long-term psychological and emotional consequences. Treatment may include psychotherapy, cognitive-behavioral therapy, and medication management.

**Social and functional consequences**

Binge eating disorder (BED) can also have various social and functional consequences that can impact an individual's quality of life. Some of these consequences include the following:

**Social isolation:** People with BED may avoid social situations, activities, or events that involve food, as they may feel embarrassed, ashamed, or guilty about their eating behaviors. As a result, it may cause sensations of seclusion and solitude.

**Impaired relationships:** BED can impact relationships with friends, family, and romantic partners. It can lead to emotional distress, arguments, and conflicts due to the individual's eating behaviors and the associated negative emotional consequences.

**Occupational impairment:** Binge eating can impact work or academic performance, leading to absenteeism, decreased productivity, and difficulty concentrating.

**Financial consequences:** BED can result in significant expenses related to food and treatment, which can impact an individual's financial stability.

**Risk of obesity-related discrimination**: People with BED who are overweight or obese may experience discrimination, stigma, and negative attitudes from others due to their weight, which can further exacerbate their emotional distress.

**Physical health consequences:** As discussed earlier, BED can lead to various physical health consequences, impacting an individual's ability to perform daily activities, work, and engage in social activities.

It is essential to seek BED treatment, as it can improve social and functional outcomes and prevent long-term negative consequences. Treatment may include psychotherapy, cognitive-behavioral therapy, medication management, and support from friends and family.

# Chapter 5:
# Treatment of BED

Treating binge eating disorder (BED) typically involves a combination of psychotherapy, medication, and lifestyle changes. The principal objectives of treatment involve mitigating episodes of binge eating, improving physical and emotional health, and improving quality of life. Some of the treatment options include:

**Cognitive-behavioral therapy (CBT):** CBT is classified as a form of psychotherapy that helps individuals change their negative thoughts and behaviors around food and body image. This therapy is often used to treat BED and can help individuals identify and challenge their binge eating triggers, develop coping skills, and learn healthy eating habits.

**Interpersonal psychotherapy (IPT):** IPT is a therapy that focuses on improving interpersonal relationships and communication skills. This therapy can help individuals with BED address any underlying interpersonal issues contributing to their binge eating behaviors.

**Medication:** Antidepressants, such as selective serotonin reuptake inhibitors (SSRIs), are sometimes used to treat BED. These drugs can aid in stabilizing mood and diminishing the frequency and severity of binge eating incidents.

**Nutrition counseling:** Working with a registered dietitian can help individuals with BED develop a healthy meal plan and learn strategies for managing cravings and binge eating behaviors.

**Lifestyle changes:** Making lifestyle changes, such as engaging in regular physical activity, practicing stress reduction techniques, and getting adequate sleep, can also help individuals with BED manage their symptoms.

Individuals with BED need to seek treatment from a mental health professional specializing in eating disorders. Treatment may involve a multidisciplinary approach that includes a team of professionals, such as a therapist, psychiatrist, dietitian, and primary care physician. With appropriate treatment, individuals with BED can improve their physical and emotional health, reduce binge eating behaviors, and improve their overall quality of life.

# Evidence-based interventions:

## Cognitive-behavioral therapy (CBT)

Cognitive-behavioral therapy (CBT) is a type of therapy that is effective in treating various mental health disorders, including binge eating disorder (BED). The underlying principle of CBT is that there is a close relationship between our thoughts, emotions, and actions and that by ch, we can improve our emotional well-being by changing our thoughts and behaviors in the context of BED; CBT typically involves identifying and challenging negative thoughts and beliefs around food and body image. This can include exploring the individual's attitudes towards their body, food, and weight and examining any patterns of thinking contributing to their binge eating behaviors.

CBT can also help individuals develop coping skills to manage cravings and the urge to binge eat. This may involve learning techniques such as mindfulness, relaxation, and distraction and developing a plan for responding to binge eating triggers.

Another important aspect of CBT for BED is developing healthy eating habits. This may involve working with a registered dietitian to create a balanced meal plan that includes all necessary nutrients. The individual may also learn strategies for managing portion sizes and healthily incorporating enjoyable foods into their diet.

CBT is typically conducted in weekly or biweekly sessions with a mental health professional specializing in eating disorders. Treatment may be individual or group-based, depending on the individual's needs and preferences.

CBT is an effective BED treatment and can help individuals reduce binge eating behaviors, improve their emotional well-being, and develop healthy habits for long-term recovery.

**Dialectical Behavior Therapy (DBT)**

Dialectical behavior therapy (DBT) was originally created to provide therapy for individuals diagnosed with Borderline Personality Disorder (BPD) but has also been found to be effective for treating other mental health conditions, including binge eating disorder (BED).

DBT is based on the idea that individuals with BED often struggle with regulating their emotions and may engage in impulsive behaviors, such as binge eating, to cope. DBT aims to help individuals develop skills to manage their feelings and reduce the urge to engage in harmful behaviors.

The therapy typically involves weekly individual therapy sessions and group skills training. The skills taught in DBT include:

**Mindfulness:** The practice of being fully present and aware of one's thoughts, feelings, and surroundings.

**Distress tolerance:** The ability to tolerate and manage difficult emotions without resorting to harmful behaviors.

**Emotion regulation:** The ability to identify and regulate intense emotions healthily.

**Interpersonal effectiveness:** The ability to communicate effectively and assertively in relationships.

DBT also emphasizes the importance of the therapeutic relationship between the client and therapist. The therapist provides validation and support while challenging negative behaviors and thought patterns.

Research has shown that DBT can effectively reduce binge eating episodes, improve mood, and increase the quality of life for individuals with BED. However, like other therapies, DBT is not a one-size-fits-all approach, and the effectiveness of the treatment can depend on factors such as individual needs and the therapist's experience.

## Interpersonal psychotherapy (IPT)

IPT is a short-term, evidence-based therapy that focuses on improving interpersonal relationships and addressing interpersonal issues contributing to mental health symptoms, including binge eating disorder (BED). The theoretical foundation of IPT is that difficulties in interpersonal relationships are at the root of psychological distress and can trigger and exacerbate psychological symptoms and that addressing these problems can improve mental health outcomes.

In IPT for BED, therapy typically involves 12-16 weekly sessions, focusing on four key problem areas: interpersonal disputes, role transitions, grief and loss, and interpersonal deficits. Through the therapeutic process, individuals work to identify specific interpersonal issues that may be contributing to their BED symptoms and develop strategies for addressing these issues constructively and effectively.

IPT may involve a range of techniques and strategies, including:

1. Encouraging open communication and expression of emotions
2. Identifying and addressing negative or maladaptive patterns of behavior in interpersonal relationships
3. Building new interpersonal skills and strategies for resolving conflicts and managing relationships.

4. Developing strategies for coping with difficult emotions and life transitions
5. Improving self-esteem and self-efficacy in interpersonal relationships

IPT effectively reduces binge eating episodes and improve overall mental health outcomes in individuals with BED. It is often combined with other treatment approaches, such as cognitive-behavioral therapy (CBT), medication, and lifestyle changes, to provide a comprehensive and individualized approach to BED treatment.

## Medication

Medication can be a helpful tool in treating binge eating disorder (BED), particularly in conjunction with other therapies such as cognitive-behavioral therapy (CBT) and nutrition counseling. However, medication is not considered a first-line treatment for BED. It is typically only prescribed in cases where other treatments have been ineffective or when an individual's symptoms are severe.

The following medications may be prescribed to treat BED:

Antidepressants: Empirical studies have demonstrated that selective serotonin reuptake inhibitors (SSRIs) and alternative antidepressants can effectively decrease instances of binge eating and enhance mood in persons diagnosed with BED. The mechanism of action of these medications involves elevating serotonin levels in the brain, which can aid in modulating mood and appetite.

Anti-seizure medications: Some anti-seizure medications, such as topiramate, have been found to reduce binge eating behaviors and promote weight loss in individuals with BED. These medications affect the brain chemicals that regulate appetite and food intake.

**Stimulants:** Stimulant medications, such as Vyvanse and Adderall (amphetamine), may be prescribed to reduce binge eating behaviors and promote weight loss in individuals with BED. These medications work by increasing levels of dopamine and norepinephrine in the brain, which can reduce appetite and food cravings.

It is crucial to emphasize that medication must always be prescribed and supervised by a medical expert and utilized alongside additional treatments such as therapy and nutritional guidance. Additionally, medication is not a BED cure, and individuals may need to continue taking medication long-term to maintain symptom control.

## Nutrition counseling

Nutrition counseling is an essential component of treatment for binge eating disorder (BED). It can help individuals develop a healthier relationship with food and learn how to nourish their bodies in a balanced and sustainable way. Nutrition counseling for BED typically involves working with a dietitian who is certified and specialized in addressing eating disorders and has expertise in helping individuals with BED.

The goals of nutrition counseling for BED may include:

1. Establishing regular and balanced meals: Individuals with BED often need help with irregular eating patterns and may skip meals or go long without eating. Nutrition counseling can help individuals establish a regular eating schedule and develop strategies for planning and preparing healthy meals.

2. Learning to recognize hunger and fullness cues: Many individuals with BED have difficulty identifying and responding to their body's hunger and fullness cues. Nutrition counseling can help individuals learn to listen to their bodies and better understand their hunger and fullness signals.

3. Developing a balanced and varied diet: Nutrition counseling can help individuals develop a diverse and balanced food that includes a variety of nutrients from all food groups. This can help individuals meet their nutrient needs, improve energy levels, and reduce cravings for high-calorie, high-fat foods.

4. Addressing disordered eating behaviors: Individuals with BED often engage in disordered eating behaviors, such as binge eating, purging, or restrictive eating. Nutrition counseling can help individuals identify and address these behaviors and develop strategies for managing them healthily and sustainably.

5. Developing a positive body image: Nutrition counseling can help individuals develop a positive and realistic body image and learn to accept and appreciate their bodies at any size.

Nutrition counseling may be provided as a standalone treatment or as part of a comprehensive treatment approach that includes other therapies and strategies for managing BED.

## Lifestyle changes

Lifestyle changes can be essential to treating individuals with binge eating disorder (BED). These changes can help promote overall health and well-being and the risk of relapse. Here are some lifestyle changes that may be recommended for individuals with BED:

**Regular exercise**: Regular physical activity can help to improve mood, reduce stress, and increase energy levels. Exercise can also help to promote weight loss and improve body image, which can be important for individuals with BED. Strive to engage in physical activity of moderate intensity, like brisk walking, for a minimum of 30 minutes or cycling, on the majority of days throughout the week.

**Balanced diet:** Eating a balanced diet that includes various foods from all the food groups may aid in lessening cravings and fostering sentiments of satiety. It is advisable to avoid missing meals, as this may result in overeating later on. Focus on eating various fruits, vegetables, whole grains, lean protein, and healthy fats.

**Mindful eating:** The concept of mindful eating revolves around being attentive to the eating experience, including the taste, texture, and aroma of food. It can help individuals with BED to develop a healthier relationship with food and reduce the risk of binge eating. Some tips for mindful eating include eating slowly, avoiding distractions (such as watching TV), and paying attention to hunger and fullness cues.

**Stress management:** Stress can trigger binge eating behaviors in some individuals. Exploring beneficial techniques for coping with stress can be useful in diminishing the likelihood of binge eating. Getting enough sleep and making time for relaxation and self-care activities are also essential.

**Support system:** Having a social network of friends and acquaintances can be beneficial in many ways. Family members or a therapist can be crucial for individuals with BED. Support can help individuals stay motivated and on track with their treatment plans and provide emotional support during difficult times.

Making lifestyle changes can be challenging, but they can be an essential part of the recovery process for individuals with BED. Working with a healthcare professional or a registered dietitian can help develop a plan tailored to an individual's needs and goals.

## Medications for BED

Currently, no medications are approved explicitly for treating binge eating disorder (BED). Nevertheless, some medications typically employed in treating various psychological disorders, such as depression and anxiety, may also be efficacious in addressing BED.

Selective serotonin reuptake inhibitors (SSRIs), an antidepressant medication, help reduce binge eating behaviors in some individuals with BED. Other antidepressant medications, such as tricyclic antidepressants and bupropion, may also be used to treat BED, although less research supports their use.

In addition to antidepressants, some individuals with BED may benefit from medications that help to regulate appetite and reduce cravings.

It's important to note that medications should be combined with psychotherapy and other behavioral interventions for BED and should only be prescribed by a healthcare provider knowledgeable about treating eating disorders.

Drugs can have side effects and may not be appropriate for all individuals with BED. A thorough evaluation and individualized treatment plan are essential for effective treatment.

## Self-help strategies and lifestyle changes

Self-help strategies and lifestyle changes can effectively reduce binge eating behaviors and improve overall well-being for individuals with binge eating disorder (BED). Here are some examples of self-help strategies and lifestyle changes that may be helpful:

Establish regular and consistent eating patterns: Eating regular, balanced meals throughout the day can help to reduce the likelihood of binge eating. It's important to avoid skipping meals or going for long periods without eating.

Keep a food diary: Keeping a record of what you eat and when you can help you identify binge eating patterns and other problematic behaviors. This can help you change your eating habits and track your progress.

**Practice mindfulness:** Mindfulness practices, such as deep breathing, meditation, and yoga, can assist in diminishing stress and anxiety, which frequently serve as triggers for binge eating. Practicing mindfulness can also help you to become more aware of your thoughts and feelings around food.

**Get regular exercise:** Exercise can help reduce and improve mood, reducing binge eating. Strive to engage in physical activity of moderate intensity for a minimum of 30 minutes most days of the week.

**Get support:** Connecting with others going through similar experiences can help reduce feelings of isolation and shame. Consider joining a support group or seeking individual therapy with a mental health professional specializing in disorders.

Avoid dieting: Restrictive diets and extreme weight loss methods can contribute to binge eating behaviors. Focus instead on developing a healthy relationship with food and your body and making sustainable lifestyle changes over time.

Self-help strategies and lifestyle changes can be essential to treating individuals with BED. It's important to work with a qualified professional knowledgeable about eating disorders to develop an individualized treatment plan that addresses your unique needs and goals.

## Support for recovery

Recovery support is essential to treat beige eating disorders (BED). Here are some examples of types of support that may be helpful:

**Support groups:** Joining a support group for individuals with eating disorders can provide a sense of community and understanding, reduce feelings of isolation and shame, and offer practical advice and encouragement.

**Family therapy:** Family therapy can help address any family dynamics that may contribute to the development or maintenance of BED. It can also provide education and support for vulnerable or overwhelmed family members.

**Individual therapy:** Individual therapy with a mental health professional specializing in eating disorders can help individuals with BED identify and address the underlying emotional and psychological factors contributing to their binge eating behaviors.

**Nutritional counseling:** Nutritional counseling with a registered dietitian can help individuals with BED to develop a healthy and balanced relationship with food. This may include creating a meal plan that provides balanced meals and snacks and learning strategies for managing cravings and urges to binge eat.

**Medication management**: For some individuals with BED, medication may help reduce the frequency and intensity of binge eating episodes. Medicines that may treat BED include antidepressants, anticonvulsants, and appetite suppressants.

**Peer support:** Connecting with others who have recovered from BED or are in recovery can provide hope, inspiration, practical advice, and encouragement.

Overall, recovery support is an integral part of the treatment of BED. Working with a healthcare professional knowledgeable about eating disorders is essential to Developing a customized plan that caters to your specific needs and objectives. And seeking support and resources to aid your recovery.

# Chapter 6:

# Recovery and Maintenance

Recovery and maintenance are crucial to fully managing binge eating disorder (BED). Recovery involves achieving a state of remission, where binge eating episodes are reduced or eliminated. However, maintaining recovery can be challenging, as people with BED may continue to experience triggers that could lead to relapse.

To maintain recovery, it is essential to continue using helpful strategies during treatment, such as practicing self-care, engaging in regular physical activity, and building a support system. It is also necessary to address any underlying emotional issues, such as anxiety or depression, as these can contribute to binge eating behavior.

In addition, maintaining a healthy relationship with food and one's body is critical for long-term recovery. This includes practicing mindful eating, which involves paying attention to hunger and fullness cues and savoring the flavors and textures of food. It also consists in cultivating a positive body image, which can be challenging in a society that often promotes unrealistic and harmful beauty standards.

Regular follow-up appointments with a healthcare provider, therapist, or nutritionist can help maintain recovery. These appointments can provide ongoing support, monitor progress, and help individuals stay accountable for their actions.

Overall, recovery and maintenance are ongoing processes that require dedication, self-awareness, and a willingness to seek help when needed. With the proper support and resources, individuals with BED can achieve long-term success and improve their overall health and well-being.

**Steps toward recovery from BED**

Recovery from binge eating disorder (BED) is a journey that may involve many steps. The following are some general stages that may be included in the recovery journey:

**Recognize and acknowledge the problem:** The first step towards recovery from BED is recognizing your problem and admitting that you need help. This may involve contacting a healthcare professional, talking to a trusted friend or family member, or joining a support group.

**Develop a treatment plan:** Once you have recognized the problem, you must have a healthcare professional knowledgeable about eating disorders to develop an individualized treatment plan that addresses your unique needs and goals. This may involve a combination of therapy, medication, and lifestyle changes.

**Address underlying emotional and psychological factors:** BED is often associated with underlying emotional and psychological factors such as stress, anxiety, depression, and low self-esteem. Addressing these factors through therapy and other techniques can help to reduce the frequency and intensity of binge eating episodes.

Develop healthy coping strategies: Healthy coping strategies for dealing with stress, anxiety, and other emotional triggers can help reduce the risk of binge eating. This may involve practicing mindfulness, regular exercise, relaxation techniques, or finding healthy ways to express your emotions.

**Learn healthy eating habits:** Learning healthy eating habits, such as eating regular meals and snacks, avoiding restrictive diets, and focusing on nutrient-dense foods, can help to reduce the risk of binge eating and promote overall physical and emotional health.

**Build a support network:** Building a support network of friends, family members, and healthcare professionals can provide the encouragement, accountability, and practical assistance needed to maintain recovery.

Overall, recovery from BED is a process that may involve many steps, setbacks, and successes. It's essential to be patient, kind, and compassionate with yourself as you work towards recovery and to seek out the support and resources you need along the way.

## Maintenance of healthy eating behaviors and a positive image

Maintaining healthy eating behaviors and a positive body image can be vital to people with binge eating disorder (BED). Here are some tips for maintaining healthy habits and a positive body image:

Follow a balanced, nutritious diet: Eating a balanced, healthy diet that includes a variety of diets to support overall physical and emotional health. It's important to avoid fad diets or restrictive eating patterns that can trigger binge eating episodes.

**Practice mindful eating:** The concept of mindful eating centers around being attentive to your sensations of hunger and fullness and eating in a relaxed, non-judgmental manner. This can help you to tune in to your body's needs and prevent overeating.

Engage in regular physical activity: Regular physical activity can help to improve mood, reduce stress, and promote overall physical health. It's important to choose activities you enjoy and is flexible rather than pushing yourself too hard or engaging in exercise as punishment.

Challenge negative body image thoughts: Negative body image thoughts can be a common feature of BED. Challenging these thoughts with positive, realistic counter-thoughts and focusing on what you appreciate about your body is essential.

**Surround yourself with supportive people:** Being with supportive people who understand your struggles and are committed to your recovery can be crucial training in healthy eating behaviors and a positive body image. This may involve joining a support group, working with a therapist or counselor, or simply spending time with friends and family who uplift and encourage you.

Overall, maintaining healthy eating behaviors and a positive body image is a process that requires ongoing effort and commitment. It's important to be kind and compassionate as you navigate the fluctuations of the healing process and seek the support and resources you need to maintain your progress.

## Relapse prevention strategies

Relapse prevention strategies can be an essential part of the recovery process for people with binge eating disorders (BED). Here are some tips for preventing relapse:

**Identify triggers:** Understanding what triggers your binge eating episodes can be crucial to preventing relapse. Keep a journal or log to track your eating habits and note any emotional or environmental triggers contributing to your binge eating.

**Develop coping strategies:** Once you've identified your triggers, it's essential to develop strategies that can help you manage stress and difficult emotions healthily. This may involve techniques such as deep breathing, meditation, or exercise.

**Practice self-care:** Self-care is integral to maintaining physical and emotional health. This may involve getting enough sleep, eating a balanced, nutritious diet, engaging in regular physical activity, and setting aside time for relaxation and leisure activities.

**Stay connected:** Maintaining social connections and a supportive network of family, friends, or peers can be crucial to preventing relapse. Stay in touch with people who understand your struggles and are committed to your recovery.

**Set realistic goals:** Setting realistic goals for yourself can help you maintain motivation and avoid feelings of disappointment or frustration contributing to relapse. Celebrate your progress and focus on the positive changes you're making.

**Seek professional support:** Finally, it's essential to seek professional help if you're struggling to maintain recovery or are experiencing persistent symptoms. Working with a therapist, counselor, or other mental health professionals can provide the necessary tools and resources to manage your symptoms and prevent relapse.

Overall, preventing relapse is a process that requires ongoing effort and commitment. It's essential to be patient and compassionate as you navigate the challenges of recovery and seek out the support and resources you need to maintain your progress.

## Support and resources for ongoing recovery

Recovery from binge eating disorder (BED) is an ongoing process that requires ongoing support and resources. Here are some resources that can be helpful for people with BED:

**Therapy and counseling:** Working with a therapist or counselor can provide ongoing support for managing symptoms, developing coping strategies, and addressing underlying psychological issues that may contribute to binge eating.

**Support groups:** Enrolling in a support group can offer a sense of camaraderie and solidarity connection with others struggling with similar issues. Support groups may be available in person or online.

**Nutrition and exercise programs:** Eating a balanced diet and engaging in regular physical activity can be critical to maintaining physical and emotional health. Community centers, gyms, or healthcare providers may offer nutrition and exercise programs.

**Self-help books and resources:** Many self-help books and online resources provide information and strategies for managing BED and related issues.

**Healthcare providers:** Working with a primary care physician, psychiatrist, or another healthcare provider can provide ongoing support and monitoring for physical and mental health issues related to BED.

**Mindfulness and meditation practices:** Mindfulness and meditation practices can help reduce and develop positive relationships with food and the body.

Overall, ongoing support and resources are critical for training in BED recovery. It's essential to seek out the help that works for your individual needs and be patient and compassionate with yourself as you navigate the ongoing challenges of recovery.

# Chapter 7:

# Personal Stories of Recovery

Personal stories of recovery from binge eating disorder (BED) can offer hope, inspiration, and practical insights into overcoming this challenging condition. Here are a few examples:

**Jenni Schaefer:** Jenni is a best-selling author, speaker, and advocate for eating disorder recovery. She struggled with BED, anorexia, and bulimia for years before seeking treatment. Through therapy, support from loved ones, and a commitment to self-care, Jenni overcame her eating disorder and built a fulfilling life in recovery. She has written several books on eating disorder recovery and speaks publicly about her experiences.

**Christy Harrison:** Christy is a registered dietitian, certified intuitive eating counselor, and host of the popular podcast "Food Psych." She also struggled with BED and other eating disorders for many years before finding recovery. Christy's approach to recovery emphasizes self-compassion, body acceptance, and a non-diet policy to nutrition. She helps others find freedom from disordered eating and body shame through her work as a counselor and educator.

**Tabitha Farrar:** Tabitha is a writer, speaker, and coach who shares her experiences recovering from BED, as well as anorexia and exercise addiction. She emphasizes the importance of challenging diet culture and societal expectations around body size and appearance. Tabitha also advocates for a non-restrictive approach to eating and encourages others to listen to their bodies hunger and fullness cues.

These are just a few examples of individuals who have successfully overcome BED and built lives of recovery. Each person's journey is unique, but these stories can offer guidance, hope, and inspiration to others struggling with this challenging condition.

## Real-life experiences of individuals with BED and their journey toward recovery

Binge eating disorder (BED) is a severe and often debilitating mental health condition that can significantly impact a person's life. However, with the proper treatment and support, overcoming BED and achieving lasting recovery is possible. Here are some real-life experiences of individuals with BED and their journey toward recovery

**Story:** Sarah had been struggling with binge eating for years. She often hid food from her family lately and felt ashamed of her behavior. After seeking help from a therapist, Sarah was diagnosed with BED and began treatment. She learned to identify and manage her triggers through therapy and develop healthier coping mechanisms. She also worked on improving her self-esteem and body image. Today, Sarah is in recovery and no longer feels controlled by her urge to binge eat.

**David's Story:** David had struggled with binge eating since childhood. He often eats to numb his anxiety and depression and feels helpless in controlling his eating habits. After reaching out for help, David was referred to a support group for individuals with BED. Through the group, he found a sense of community and understanding that he had never experienced before. He also learned practical strategies for managing his binge eating, such as mindfulness and distraction techniques. Today, David is in recovery and regularly attends support group meetings.

**Maria's Story:** Maria had been struggling with BED for several years when she reached a breaking point. She had gained an insignificant and was experiencing health problems due to binge eating. After seeking help from a nutritionist and therapist, Maria began making lifestyle changes to support her recovery. She started exercising regularly and eating a balanced diet and worked on improving her relationship with food.

With the support of her healthcare team and loved ones, Maria overcame her binge eating and achieved lasting recovery.

The aforementioned instances are merely a few of the numerous possibilities for individuals who have recovered from BED. Recovery is a unique journey for each person, and it may involve a combination of therapies and lifestyle changes. The key is to seek help and support and to stay committed to the recovery process. Overcoming BED and leading a fulfilling, healthy life is possible with time and effort.

## Lessons learned and insights for others with BED

Individuals with binge eating disorder (BED) who have successfully overcome the disease have shared some valuable lessons and insights for others who may be struggling with BED:

**Seek help:** The first step towards recovery is seeking help. It takes courage to reach out for assistance, but it is necessary to get the proper treatment.

**Address underlying emotional issues:** BED is often linked to underlying emotional problems, such as depression, anxiety, and low self-esteem. Addressing these issues is crucial for successful recovery.

**Practice self-compassion:** BED can be a source of shame and guilt, perpetuating the binge eating cycle. Practicing self-compassion and forgiving oneself for past behaviors is essential.

**Identify triggers and develop coping mechanisms:** It is important to identify triggers that lead to binge eating and develop healthy coping mechanisms to deal with them.

Build a support system: Recovery from BED can be challenging, and having a supportive network can make a significant difference. Joining a support group or seeking help from friends and family can provide the necessary support.

**Focus on progress, not perfection:** Recovery from BED is a continuous process that requires time and effort. It is essential to focus on improvement rather than perfection and celebrate every small achievement.

Embrace a healthy lifestyle: Adopting a healthy lifestyle, including regular exercise and a balanced diet, can benefit physical and mental health.

**Stay committed to recovery:** BED recovery is a lifelong process, and staying committed to recovery is essential. Consistently practicing healthy behaviors and seeking ongoing support can help maintain recovery.

# Chapter 8:
# Future Directions and Research

Future directions and research in binge eating disorder (BED) are vital for advancing our understanding of the disorder and improving treatment options. Here are some notes on potential future directions and research areas:

**Treatment improvement:** More research is needed to determine the most effective approaches for treating BED, especially given the frequent comorbidity of other mental health conditions, such as depression or anxiety, in adolescents, men, and older adults. Additionally, more research is required to determine the best way to deliver treatment, such as through telehealth or group therapy.

**Prevention:** Prevention efforts for BED are limited. Future research could explore developing and implementing prevention programs targeting individuals at risk for developing BED.

Comorbid conditions: BED often co-occurs with other mental health conditions, such as depression and anxiety. Future research could explore the relationship between BED and these comorbid conditions and identify the most effective treatments for individuals with both conditions.

**Neurobiological factors:** There is growing evidence that neurobiological factors play a role in developing and maintaining BED. Future research could further explore these factors and identify potential targets for treatment.

**Genetics:** Genetic factors may contribute to the development of BED. More research is needed to identify specific genes and genetic pathways associated with BED.

**Sociocultural factors:** Sociocultural factors, such as weight stigma and social media, may contribute to the development of BED. Future research could explore the relationship between these factors and BED and identify potential interventions.

**Long-term outcomes:** Research on the long-term consequences of BED treatment is limited. Future research could explore the long-term effects of therapy on binge eating behavior, weight, and other health outcomes.

Overall, future directions and research in BED are critical for advancing our understanding of the disorder and improving treatment options.

## Current challenges and gaps in understanding BED

Despite the growing recognition of binge eating disorder (BED) as a severe mental health condition, several challenges and gaps in understanding BED need to be addressed. Some of these challenges and gaps include:

**Lack of awareness:** Many people, including healthcare providers, are unaware of BED, which can lead to misdiagnosis or lack of appropriate treatment.

**Stigma and shame:** BED is often stigmatized, and people with BED may feel ashamed and reluctant to seek help.

**Limited research:** Compared to other eating disorders, there is relatively little research on BED, and more research is needed to understand its causes, risk factors, and effective treatments.

**Lack of standardized diagnostic criteria:** While BED is acknowledged as a separate condition in the DSM-5, there still needs to be more clarity over its diagnostic criteria, which can lead to inconsistencies in diagnosis and treatment.

**Limited access to treatment:** Despite the high prevalence of BED, there is still limited access to evidence-based therapies, such as CBT, IPT, and medication.

**Co-occurring conditions:** Numerous individuals with BED also encounter other psychological conditions, including depression or anxiety, which can complicate diagnosis and treatment.

**Cultural considerations:** Cultural factors, such as body image ideals, can impact the development and treatment of BED, and more research is needed to understand these factors.

Addressing these challenges and gaps in understanding BED will require a coordinated effort from healthcare providers, researchers, and policymakers. This can include increasing awareness of BED, reducing stigma, expanding access to evidence-based treatments, and addressing cultural factors that impact the development and treatment of BED.

# Chapter 9:
# Conclusion

In conclusion, Binge Eating Disorder (BED) is a serious and complex eating disorder that affects individuals physically, emotionally, and mentally. It can lead to a range of health complications, including obesity, heart disease, and mental health disorders. However, with appropriate treatment and support, recovery from BED is possible. Treatment may include psychotherapy, medication, nutritional counseling, and lifestyle changes, such as exercise and stress management techniques.

Individuals with BED need to seek professional help and develop a personalized treatment plan that addresses their unique needs and goals. Loved ones can also play a vital role in supporting individuals with BED by educating themselves about the disorder, providing emotional support, and encouraging them to seek treatment.

# Summary of key points

Binge Eating Disorder (BED) is a mental health condition characterized by recurrent episodes of binge eating.

BED is associated with physical and mental health risks, including obesity, cardiovascular problems, and depression.

BED treatment often involves a combination of therapy, medication, and lifestyle changes, such as mindful eating and regular physical activity.

Support from loved ones and a sense of community can be beneficial for individuals with BED.

Further research is necessary to determine the most effective treatments for BED and to better understand the underlying causes of the disorder.

# Final thoughts and recommendations for individuals with BED and their loved ones

Seek professional help: Binge eating disorder is a serious condition that requires professional help. Consider seeing a therapist, psychiatrist, registered dietitian, or other healthcare professionals who specialize in treating eating disorders.

Create a support system: Surround yourself with a supportive network of family and friends who understand and can offer encouragement and support.

Practice self-care: Self-care is important in managing binge eating disorder. This can include engaging in regular physical activity, getting enough sleep, practicing, and taking time for self-care activities that you enjoy.

Focus on a balanced diet: It's important to eat a balanced diet that includes a variety of nutrient-dense foods. Avoid skipping meals or severely restricting your intake, as this can trigger binge episodes.

Mindful eating: Practice mindful eating by paying attention to your hunger and fullness cues, savoring your food, and eating without distractions.

Avoid triggers: Identify your triggers and avoid them as much as possible. This may include certain foods, situations, or emotions that may lead to binge episodes.

Stay positive: Recovery from a binge eating disorder is a journey, and it may take time to see progress. Stay positive and focus on the small victories along the way.

Remember, you are not alone in your journey to recovery. With the right treatment and support, it is possible to overcome a binge eating disorder and lead a fulfilling life.